FAINTING
AND
SYNCOPE SYNDROME

By:

Kevin R. Sweeter

Contents

Introduction — Page 1

What is Syncope Syndrome? — Page 3

Types of Syncope — Page 5

What are the Causes and Symptoms — Page 7

Diagnosis — Page 27

First Aid / Treatment — Page 21

Possible Prevention Measures — Page 37

Author's Note — Page 39

Introduction

Fainting is a problem, and not just from the physical problems that may be associated with episodes or occurrences, but it also defeats the fundamental fight - or – flight instinct that could save a life in times of extreme need or danger.

Like a person who just stands there screaming during an emergency situation, a fainter is actually more of a liability than a hindrance, or help.

Though typical fainting spells only last a few seconds to mere minutes, I a crisis where every moment counts, this can be rather fatal.

Then there is also the potential fall injury as a result of fainting, whereby someone could get seriously hurt.

The elderly and women seem to experience fainting the most.

What causes a person to faint?

What are the symptoms of fainting?

How is fainting diagnosed?

Is fainting preventable?

Is fainting curable?

Follow along now and read about the mechanisms and causes of fainting, the diagnostic procedures and possible warning signs and what to do with someone who faints.

What is Syncope Syndrome?

Syncope, pronounced Sin-koa-pee, is a temporary loss of consciousness usually related to insufficient blood flow to the brain, occurring most often when blood pressure is too low, also called hypotension, and the heart doesn't pump enough oxygen to the brain.

It can be benign or a symptom of an underlying medical condition.

What is Fainting?

The Loss of consciousness for a short time because of a temporarily insufficient supply of oxygen to the brain.

Also known as to pass out, lose consciousness, black out, keel over, swoon.

Fainting, also called syncope, is a sudden, brief loss of consciousness and posture caused by decreased blood flow to the brain.

Types of Syncope

Vasovagal syncope

Also called **cardio-neurogenic syncope**.

Vasovagal syncope is the most common type of syncope.

It may also be called **neurocardiogenic** syncope.

Neurocardiogenic syncope, also called the common faint or **vasovagal syncope**, occurs in about 25 to 40 percent of the people who have syncope. These fainting episodes are related to problems with both the heart and the nervous system.

Vasovagal syncope occurs when you faint because your body overreacts to certain triggers, such as the sight of blood or under an extreme emotional distress.

The vasovagal syncope trigger causes your heart rate and blood pressure to drop suddenly.

Situational syncope

Is the temporary loss of consciousness in a particular kind of situation. The situations that can trigger this reaction are diverse, and include such things as having blood drawn, straining while urinating or defecating, and even during coughing fits. It can also be triggered due to the emotional stress, extreme fear, or pain experienced during an unexpected or unusual situation.

Postural syncope, also called **postural hypotension**, is a transient loss of consciousness secondary to a reduction in cerebral blood flow, and is typically precipitated by standing up too fast.

It is the most common cause of **recurrent transient** loss of consciousness.

Neurologic syncope

Neurologic syncope is related to problems with the nervous system, such as seizures. Often perhaps accompanying an epileptic seizure.

Postural Orthostatic Tachycardia Syndrome (POTS)

Also referred to as **POTS** and is one of a group of disorders that have **orthostatic intolerance** or OI, as their **primary symptom**. OI describes a condition in which an excessively reduced volume of blood returns to the heart after an individual stands up from a lying down position.

Unknown Causes of Syncope

In a large number of cases of fainting, the cause is unknown, which is making the proper diagnoses and treatment decisions to become more difficult.

Current ongoing research indicates no known physical or neurological causes at work in these cases, which continues to baffle researchers.

What are the Causes and Symptoms?

With fainting or syncope, the patient is unaware that they have passed out and fallen to the ground. It is only after the episode that they understand what has happened.

There may be symptoms or signs before the episode, which may include:

The person may feel lightheaded, nauseated, sweaty, or weak. There may be a feeling of dizziness or vertigo such as with the room spinning, vision may fade or blur, and there may be muffled hearing and tingling sensations in the body.

With pre-syncope or a near faint, the same symptoms will occur, but the person doesn't quite lose consciousness.

During the fainting episode, when the person is unconscious, there may a few twitches of the body, which may be confused with seizure activity.

The person may have some confusion after wakening but it should resolve within a few seconds.

After a fainting episode, there should be a quick return to normal mental function, though there may be other signs and symptoms depending upon the underlying cause or causes of the faint. An example would be if the individual is in the midst of a heart attack, he or she might complain of chest pain or pressure.

Many different conditions can cause fainting. These include heart problems such as irregular heartbeats, seizures, low blood sugar, or hypoglycemia, anemia, which is a deficiency in healthy oxygen carrying cells, and problems with how the nervous system, or the body's system of nerves, which regulates blood pressure. Some types of fainting seems to run in families.

While fainting may indicate a particular medical condition, sometimes it may occur in an otherwise healthy individual.

Fainting is a particular problem for the elderly who may suffer serious injuries from falls when they faint. Most episodes are very brief, and in most cases, the individual who has fainted regains complete consciousness within just a few minutes.

Fainting is a common problem, accounting for some 3 percent of emergency room visits and 6 percent of hospital admissions. It can happen in otherwise healthy people. A person may feel faint and lightheaded, also called presyncope, or lose consciousness, syncope, altogether.

Fainting may have a variety of causes. A simple episode, also called a vasovagal attack or neurally-mediated syncope, is the most common type of fainting spell. It is most common in children and young adults. A vasovagal attack happens because blood pressure drops, reducing circulation to the brain and causing loss of consciousness.

Typically, an attack occurs while standing and is often preceded by a sensation of warmth, nausea, lightheadedness, and a form of visual gray out.

If the syncope is prolonged, it can trigger an actual seizure.

You may suffer from a simple fainting spell due to anxiety, fear, pain, intense emotional stress, hunger, or use of alcohol or drugs. Most people who suffer from simple fainting have no underlying heart or neurological, or nerve or brain, problems.

Some people have a problem with the way their body regulates their blood pressure, particularly when they move too quickly from a lying or sitting position to a standing position. This condition is called postural hypotension and may be severe enough to cause fainting.

This type of fainting is more common in the elderly, people who recently had a lengthy illness that kept them in bed and people who have poor muscle tone.

Diseases of the autonomic nervous system. Your autonomic nervous system is the part of the nervous system that controls involuntary vital functions, such as the beating of your heart, the degree to which your blood vessels are constricted, and breathing.

Autonomic nervous system problems include acute or subacute dysautonomia, chronic post-ganglionic autonomic insufficiency, and chronic pre-ganglionic autonomic insufficiency. If you have one of these disorders, you are likely to have other symptoms, such as erectile dysfunction, or the inability to have or maintain an erection, loss of bladder and bowel control, loss of the normal reflexes of your pupils, or decreased sweating, tearing, and salivation.

Conditions that interfere with the parts of the nervous system that regulate blood pressure and heart rate.

These conditions include: diabetes, alcoholism, malnutrition, and amyloidosis, in which waxy protein builds up in the tissues and organs. If you take certain high blood pressure drugs, which act on your blood vessels, you may be more likely to suffer from fainting. If you are dehydrated, which may affect the amount of blood in your body and, thus, your blood pressure, you may be more likely to faint.

Heart or blood vessel problems that interfere with blood flow to the brain.

These may include heart block, or a problem with the electrical impulses that control your heart muscle

Problems with the sinus node, a specialized area of your heart that helps it beat

Heart arrhythmia, or an irregular heart rhythm

A blood clot in the lungs

An abnormally narrowed aortic heart valve, or certain other problems with the structure of your heart.

Conditions that may cause unusual patterns of stimulation to particular nerves.

These include micturition syncope, or fainting during or after urination

Glossopharyngeal neuralgia, or fainting due to inflammation and pain in a particular nerve to the mouth

Cough syncope, or fainting after intense coughing

Stretch syncope, or fainting that occurs when stretching the neck and arms.

Hyperventilation.

If you become intensely anxious or panicked and breathe too quickly, you may feel faint from hyperventilation, or the act of taking in too much oxygen and getting rid of too much carbon dioxide too quickly.

Being unconscious is not normal; those affected should seek medical care.

• Syncope may be caused by a variety of mechanisms, but isn't caused by head injury, which is considered a concussion.

• Some causes of syncope can be a warning of a life-threatening situation. Most times, syncope is a relatively benign situation.

• While most episodes of syncope can be easily explained, some patients never receive a diagnosis or know the specific cause.

Fainting, blacking out, or syncope, is the temporary loss of consciousness followed by the return to full wakefulness. This loss of consciousness may be accompanied by loss of muscle tone that can result in falling or slumping over. To better understand why fainting can occur; it is helpful to explain why somebody is awake.

The brain has multiple parts, including two hemispheres, the cerebellum, and the brain stem. The brain requires blood flow to provide oxygen and glucose, or sugar, to its cells to sustain life. The liver typically provides the glucose to the body.

For the body to be awake, an area known as the reticular activating system located in the brain stem needs to be turned on, and at least one brain hemisphere needs to be functioning.

For fainting or syncope to occur, either the reticular activating system loses its blood supply, or both hemispheres of the brain are deprived of blood, oxygen, or glucose. If blood sugar levels are normal, blood flow must be briefly disrupted to the whole brain or to the reticular activating system for fainting to occur.

Fainting is not caused by head trauma.

Since loss of consciousness after a head injury is considered a concussion., however, fainting can cause injury if the person falls and hurts themselves, or if the faint occurs while participating in an activity like driving a car.

Fainting is differentiated from seizure, during which patients may also lose consciousness.

Decreased blood flow to the brain can occur because:

The heart fails to pump the blood

The blood vessels don't have enough tone to maintain blood pressure to deliver the blood to the brain

There is not enough blood or fluid within the blood vessels

In the past when clothing like corsets were commonly used, restriction of blood flow throughout the body was a common cause of fainting. That is why such furnishings known as fainting couches were created.

A combination of one or more of these conditions listed above.

Heart rhythm changes

Heart rhythm changes are the most common causes of passing out, fainting, or syncope.

While this may sound ominous, frequently the faint is due to a temporary, but brief change in normal body function.

Sometimes, the heart rhythm change is more dangerous and potentially life-threatening.

The heart is an electrical pump, and if an electrical system problem exists, the heart may on occasion be unable to adequately pump blood, causing short-term drops in blood pressure. The electrical issues may cause the heart to beat too quickly, too slowly, or erratically.

A rapid heart rate or tachycardia

Is an abnormal rhythm generated in either the upper or lower chambers of the heart and may be life-threatening.

Should the heart beat too quickly, there may not be enough time for it to fill with blood in between each heartbeat, which then decreases the amount of blood the heart can deliver to the body. Tachycardias can occur at any age and may not be related to atherosclerotic heart disease.

With bradycardia, or a slow heart rate, the heart's ability to pump blood may be compromised. As the heart ages, the electrical system can become fragile and heart blocks, or disruptions of the electrical system, can occur, causing the heart rate to slow down.

Aside from structural electrical problems with the heart, medications may be the culprit.

When taking prescribed medications especially for blood pressure control.

Beta blockers such as:

Metoprolol, or Lopressor, Toprol XL

Propranolol, or Inderal, Inderal LA

Atenolol, or Tenormin

Calcium channel blockers such as:

Diltiazem, or Cardizem, Dilacor, Tiazac

Verapamil, or Calan, Verelan and others

Amlodipine, or Norvasc

The heart can become more sensitive to the effects of these drugs and beat abnormally slow, decreasing blood output from the heart.

Heart structural conditions

Structural problems with the heart can cause fainting or syncope, either because there is a problem with the ability of the heart to adequately pump blood or because of valve problems.

When the heart muscle becomes damaged or inflamed it may not have the ability to pump blood to meet the body's needs.

Examples of this include a heart attack, or myocardial infarction, or cardiomyopathy, in which the heart muscle weakens.

Heart valve conditions

Abnormalities with the heart valves can also cause fainting or syncope. The valves allow blood to go in the proper direction when the heart pumps. Valve diseases may include abnormal narrowing, or stenosis, or leakage, or insufficiency or regurgitation.

Either situation can cause issues with maintaining adequate blood flow to the body.

Sudden cardiac death

In young people, especially athletes, fainting, or syncope can occur because of abnormal thickening of parts of the heart muscle, also called hypertrophic cardiomyopathy.

This condition may obstruct blood when it tries to leave the heart, especially when the heart is asked to beat harder during exercise.

Sudden death in athletes may be foreshadowed by episodes of syncope.

Postural hypotension

Loss of intravascular fluid, that is the blood and water within the blood vessels, can also cause fainting or syncope.

Usually, fainting will occur when a person stands up quickly from a lying or sitting position and there isn't enough time for the body to compensate by making the heart beat quicker, or having the blood vessels constrict to maintain the body's blood pressure and blood flow to the brain.

This is referred to aspostural hypotension.

Vasovagal syncope

Vasovagal syncope is one of the most common causes of fainting. In this situation, the balance between the chemicals adrenaline and acetylcholine is greatly disrupted.

Adrenaline stimulates the body.

Including making the heart beat faster and blood vessels narrower, adrenaline thereby increases blood pressure.

Acetylcholine does the opposite.

When the vagus nerve is stimulated, excess acetylcholine is released, the heart rate slows, and the blood vessels dilate, making it harder for blood to defeat gravity and be pumped to the brain. This temporary decrease in blood flow to the brain and causes the syncope, or fainting episode.

Pain can stimulate the vagus nerve and is a common cause of vasovagal syncope.

Other noxious stimuli can do the same thing, including situational stressors.

It is common for medical and nursing students to faint when observing their first operation or autopsy. Some people pass out when they hear bad news; others may pass out when they experience the sight of blood or needles.

In the Victorian age, this was known as a swoon.

Other situations commonly cause the heart rate to temporarily slow and cause a faint.

Straining with urination, bowel movement, or coughing can cause a vagal response, an increase in acetylcholine levels, and or a decrease in blood flow to the brain.

Anemia, or low red blood cell count, whether it occurs acutely from bleeding or gradually for a variety of reasons, can cause fainting because there aren't enough red blood cells to deliver oxygen to the brain.

Dehydration, or lack of water in the body can similarly cause fainting or syncope. This can be caused by excessive loss of water from vomiting, diarrhea, sweating, or by inadequate fluid intake.

Some illnesses like diabetes can cause dehydration by excess loss of water in the urine.

Orthostatic hypotension

Blood vessels need to maintain their tone so that the body can withstand the effects of gravity with changes in position.

When the body position changes from lying down to standing, the autonomic nervous system, or the part of the brain not under conscious control, increases tone in the blood vessel walls, making them constrict, and at the same time increasing the heart rate so that blood can be pumped upward to the brain.

As people age, blood vessels may become less resilient, and orthostatic hypotension, or relative low blood pressure with standing, may occur and cause syncope.

Vertebrobasilar Artery Disease

Blood vessels to the brain are no different from any other blood vessels in the body and are at risk for narrowing with age.

Smoking, high blood pressure, high cholesterol, and diabetes all can contribute to narrowing of blood vessels.

While most people are aware of the carotid arteries that supply the thinking parts of the brain, another set of arteries supply the base of the brain.

This vertebrobasilar system is also at risk for narrowing, and should there be a temporary disruption in the blood flow to the midbrain and the reticular activating system, fainting or syncope may occur.

The vertebral arteries run to the brain in the back of the neck and are encased in bony tunnels. If blood flow in these arteries is disrupted for any reason, the brain stem and reticular activating system may turn off, causing syncope.

Electrolyte imbalance

Electrolyte and hormone abnormalities may also be responsible for syncope; however, these causes are due to their effects on the heart and blood vessels.

Other medications and drugs

Other medications or drugs may also be potential causes of fainting or syncope including those for **high blood pressure** that can dilate blood vessels, **antidepressants** that can affect heart electrical activity, and those that affect mental status like **pain medications, alcohol**, and **cocaine.**

Pregnancy

Syncope is also related to pregnancy.

Likely explanations include compression of the inferior vena cava, or the large vein that returns blood to the heart by the enlarging uterus and by orthostatic hypotension.

Deglutition, or Swallowing, syncope

Syncope may occur during deglutition.

Deglutition syncope is characterized by loss of consciousness on swallowing

It has been associated not only with ingestion of solid food, but also with carbonated and ice-cold beverages, and even with belching.

Cardiac Conditions

Syncope from Bradycardia

Cardiac arrhythmias

The most common cause of cardiac syncope is cardiac arrhythmia, or abnormal heart rhythm, wherein the heart beats too slowly, too rapidly, or too irregularly to pump enough blood to the brain.

Some arrhythmias can be life-threatening.

Two major groups of arrhythmias are bradycardia and tachycardia.

Bradycardia can be caused by heart blocks.

Tachycardias include SVT, or supraventricular tachycardia and VT, or ventricular tachycardia.

SVT does not cause syncope except in Wolff-Parkinson-White syndrome. Ventricular tachycardia originate in the ventricles. VT causes syncope and can result in sudden death. Ventricular tachycardia, which describes a heart rate of over 100 beats per minute with at least three irregular heartbeats as a sequence of consecutive premature beats, can degenerate into ventricular fibrillation, which is rapidly fatal without cardiopulmonary resuscitation, or CPR, and defibrillation.

Typically, tachycardic-generated syncope is caused by a cessation of beats following a tachycardic episode. This condition, called tachycardia-bradycardia syndrome, is usually caused by sinoatrial node dysfunction or block or atrioventricular block.

Obstructive cardiac lesion

Aortic stenosis and mitral stenosis are the most common examples. Aortic stenosis presents with repeated episodes of syncope.

A pulmonary embolism can cause obstructed blood vessels and is the cause of syncope in less than 1 percent of people who present to the emergency department.

Rarely, cardiac tumors such as atrial myxomas can also lead to syncope.

Structural cardiopulmonary disease

These are relatively infrequent causes of fainting.

The most common cause in this category is fainting associated with an acute myocardial infarction or ischemic event.

The faint in this case is primarily caused by an abnormal nervous system reaction similar to the reflex faints. In general, faints caused by structural disease of the heart or blood vessels are particularly important to recognize, as they are warning of potentially life-threatening conditions.

Among other conditions prone to trigger syncope, by either hemodynamic compromise or by a neural reflex mechanism, or both, some of the most important are hypertrophic cardiomyopathy, acute aortic dissection, pericardial tamponade, pulmonary embolism, aortic stenosis, and pulmonary hypertension.

Other cardiac causes

Sick sinus syndrome, a sinus node dysfunction, causing alternating bradycardia and tachycardia. Often there is a long pause asystole between heartbeat.

Adams-Stokes syndrome is a cardiac syncope that occurs with seizures caused by complete or incomplete heart block. Symptoms include deep and fast respiration, weak and slow pulse and respiratory pauses that may last for 60 seconds.

Subclavian steal syndrome arises from retrograde (reversed) flow of blood in the vertebral artery or the internal thoracic artery, due to a proximal stenosis, or narrowing and / or occlusion of the subclavian artery.

Aortic dissection, or a tear in the aorta, and cardiomyopathy can also result in syncope.

Surgery

Healthy individuals may experience minor symptoms, such as lightheadedness, greying-out as they experience surgery or the recovery thereafter, or other physical trauma not related to life threatening situations. Much like as with watching your blood being drawn, or observing an open wound syncope can occur.

Other causes

Factors that influence fainting are fasting for long hours, or especially for days, taking in too little food and fluids, low blood pressure, hypoglycemia, high g-force, emotional distress, and lack of sleep.

One theory in evolutionary psychology is that fainting at the sight of blood might have evolved as a form of playing dead which increased survival from attackers and might have slowed blood loss in a primitive environment.

Blood-injury phobia, as this is called, is experienced by about 15 percent of people.

Fainting can occur in cough syncope following severe fits of coughing, such as that associated with pertussis or whooping cough.

Diagnosis

A complete blood count, or CBC, test, electrocardiogram and tilt-table test are some of the procedures used to diagnose fainting, or syncope.

As with most medical conditions, the history is the key in finding out why a patient faints.

Since most episodes of syncope do not occur while the patient is wearing a heart monitor in front of a medical provider, it is the description of how the patient felt and what bystanders or family members witnessed that will give clues to the diagnosis.

Physical examination will try to look for signs that will give direction to the potential diagnosis. Heart monitoring may be done to look for heart rhythm disturbances. Blood pressure may be checked, both while lying and standing to uncover orthostatic hypotension. Examination of the heart, lung, and neurologic system may uncover a potential cause if these are abnormal.

Initial diagnostic tests may include an electrocardiogram, or EKG, and screening blood tests like a complete blood count, or CBC, electrolytes, glucose, and kidney function tests. Thyroid blood tests may also be performed.

Heart rhythm disturbances may be transient and not always evident at time of the examination. On occasion, a heart monitor, or Holter monitor, can be worn as an outpatient for 24 or 48 hours or for up to 30 days, or also known as an event monitor. Abnormal heart rhythms and rates may be uncovered as the potential cause of syncope.

A tilt-table test can be used to uncover orthostatic hypotension and is usually done on an outpatient basis.

This is where the patient is placed at an angle on a table for 30 to 45 minutes, and blood pressure and pulse rate are measured with the patient in different positions.

Depending upon the suspicions of the health care provider, imaging may be done of the brain using computerized tomography, or CT scan, or with a magnetic resonance imaging, or MRI.

Often these tests are normal and a presumptive diagnosis is made of a non-life-threatening event. However, the medical care provider may decide, in consultation with the patient, whether further testing is required and whether testing should occur in the hospital or as an outpatient.

It may be reasonable in some cases to take a watchful waiting approach and not proceed with any further evaluation.

Diagnostic approach

A hemoglobin count may indicate anemia or blood loss. However, this has been useful in only about 5 percent of patients evaluated for fainting.

An electrocardiogram, or ECG, records the electrical activity of the heart. It is estimated that from 20 percent to 50 percent of patients have an abnormal ECG. However, while an ECG may identify conditions such as atrial fibrillation, heart block, or a new or old heart attack, it typically does not provide a definite diagnosis for the underlying cause for fainting.

For people with more than two episodes of syncope and no diagnosis on routine testing, an insertable cardiac monitor might be used. It lasts 28 to 36 months.

Smaller than a pack of gum, it is inserted just beneath the skin in the upper chest area. The procedure typically takes 15 to 20 minutes. Once inserted, the device continuously monitors the rate and rhythm of the heart. Upon waking from a fainting spell, the patient places a hand held pager-sized device called an Activator over the implanted device and simply presses a button.

This information is stored and retrieved by their physician and some devices can be monitored remotely.

Imaging

For people with uncomplicated syncope, that is one without seizures and a normal neurological exam, computed tomography or MRI is not generally indicated.

Likewise, using carotid ultrasonography on the premise of identifying carotid artery disease as a cause of syncope also is not indicated. Although sometimes investigated as a cause of syncope, carotid artery problems are unlikely to cause that condition.

San Francisco syncope rule

The San Francisco syncope rule was developed to isolate people who have higher risk for a serious cause of syncope.

High risk is anyone who has:

Congestive heart failure, hematocrit of <30 percent

Electrocardiograph abnormality

Shortness of breath

Or a systolic blood pressure of <90 mmHg

The San Francisco syncope rule however was not validated by subsequent studies.

Society and culture

Fainting in women was a commonplace trope or stereotype in Victorian England and in contemporary and modern depictions of the period.

This may have been partly due to genuine ill health, or the respiratory effects of corsets are frequently cited, but it was fashionable for women to affect an aristocratic frailty

and create a scene by fainting at a dramatic moment. Or
fake fainting.

Falling-out is a culture-bound syndrome primarily
reported in the southern United States and the Caribbean.

Some individuals occasionally or frequently play the
fainting game, also referred to in the US as the choking
game, which involves the deliberate induction of syncope
via voluntary restriction of blood flow to the brain, an
action that can result in acute or cumulative brain damage
and even death.

First Aid / Treatment

Fainting is not normal, although the cause may not be serious, but when in doubt, calling 911, activating the emergency medical system, and seeking medical care is appropriate.

It is always appropriate to seek medical care.

If the episode is short-lived and the person returns to normal function with no evidence of injury, it may be appropriate to contact the primary care practitioner to discuss care options.

If the person is not breathing and no pulse can be felt or detected, 911 should be activated, an AED, or an automated external defibrillator, placed, and bystander CPR should be initiated.

In the ambulance, hospital, or doctor's office, because the potential life-threatening causes of syncope need to be initially considered; often a patient who complains of fainting, or syncope, will be placed on a heart monitor, have an intravenous line placed, and oxygen supplied.

A finger stick blood sugar may be checked to look for hypoglycemia, or low blood sugar.

Further treatment will be tailored to the specific cause of the fainting or syncope based upon the patient's evaluation.

What to do with a person who has fainted

Position the person on his or her back.

If there are no injuries and the person is breathing, raise the person's legs above heart level — about 12 inches, if possible.

Loosen belts, collars or other constrictive clothing.

To reduce the chance of fainting again, don't get the person up too quickly.

Management

Recommended acute treatment of vasovagal and orthostatic, or hypotension, syncope involves returning blood to the brain by positioning the person on the ground, with legs slightly elevated or leaning forward and the head between the knees for at least 10–15 minutes, preferably in a cool and quiet place.

For individuals who have problems with chronic fainting spells, therapy should focus on recognizing the triggers and learning techniques to keep from fainting.

At the appearance of warning signs such as lightheadedness, nausea, or cold and clammy skin, counter-pressure maneuvers that involve gripping fingers into a fist, tensing the arms, and crossing the legs or squeezing the thighs together can be used to ward off a fainting spell.

Once the symptoms have passed, sleep is recommended.

If fainting spells occur often without a triggering event, syncope may be a sign of an underlying heart disease. In case syncope is caused by cardiac disease, the treatment is much more sophisticated than that of vasovagal syncope and may involve pacemakers and implantable cardioverter-defibrillators depending on the precise cardiac cause.

Possible Preventive Measures

Depending upon the cause, there may be opportunity to prevent fainting spells.

For example:

Patients who have had a vasovagal episode may be aware of the warning signs and be able to sit or lie down before passing out and avert the fainting episode.

For older patients with orthostatic hypotension, waiting for a second after changing positions may be all that is needed to allow the body's reflexes to react.

Medications may be adjusted if they are thought to be the potential cause of fainting or syncope.

Adequate fluid intake may be enough to prevent dehydration as the cause for syncope.

There is an increased awareness of syncope and sudden death in younger athletes due to hypertrophic cardiomyopathy.

A variety of screening tests are available to assess potential risk for sudden death, but no consensus yet as to who and when to screen athletes has emerged.

Fainting doesn't have to interfere with your life, it can be controlled or even prevented. With awareness and caution, proper procedures, and care, fainting can indeed be regulated and managed effectively.

Author's Note:

I thank you for your patronage and hope that you enjoy your new book! Reviews are encouraged; please feel free to share your experience with others.
~Kevin R. Sweeter

Follow on my Amazon Author Page:

https://www.amazon.com/Kevin-R.Sweeter/e/B00500O7U4

Keep up to date with availability and promotions.

Contact E-mail: kevin.r.sweeter.author@gmail.com

Please subscribe to my author email list for news, updates, and special offers and events.

Like, Follow, and Share on my Facebook Author Page:

https://www.facebook.com/Kevin-Sweeter-Author-209756967060/

Visit the book pages; see what is in the works, what is published, what will come soon, and what the books are about. Invite your friends to 'like' my pages.